Kettlebell Training for Beginners

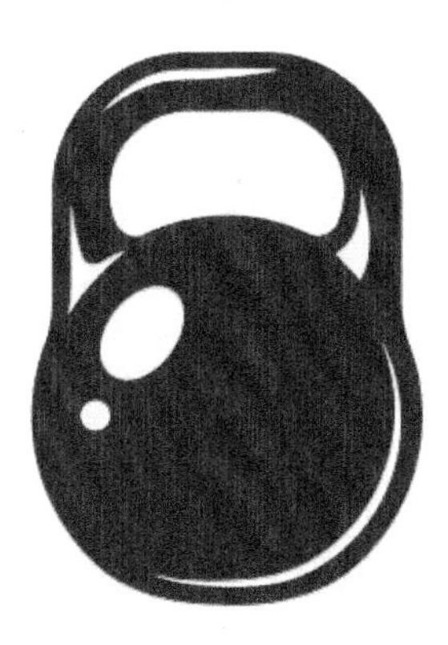

By Whit McClendon

Also by Whit McClendon

Short Workouts For Beginners:
Get Healthier and Stronger at Home

More Beginner Workouts: The Next Step
Training at Home with Basic Equipment

Kettlebell Training for Beginners

The Basics: Swings, Snatches, Get Ups, and More

Book 3 in the Jade Mountain Workout Series

By Whit McClendon

Copyrights

Kettlebell Training for Beginners
The Basics: Swings, Snatches, Get Ups, and More

Disclaimer:

The material contained in this book is for informational purposes only. The author and anyone else affiliated with the creation or distribution of this book may not be held liable for damages of any kind whatsoever allegedly caused or resulting from any person performing the workouts and exercises depicted herein. Before beginning this or any other workout routine, it is recommended that you consult with your physician for authorization and clearance. If you have problems with your health, you should seek clearance from a qualified medical professional. The information contained here in is not intended to, and never should, substitute for the necessity of seeking the advice of a qualified medical professional. If at any time you feel pain or discomfort, stop immediately.

ISBN-13: 978-1-7326300-3-1 (Rolling Scroll Publishing)
ISBN-10: 1-7326300-3-8

Cover Art by: Whit McClendon
Published by: ~~Jade Mountain Martial Arts, Inc./Rolling~~
Scroll Publishing, Katy, TX
Website: www.jmma.org

Table of Contents

Acknowledgements

I've been learning and teaching martial arts and fitness concepts for over 30 years. Not only has it been exceedingly fun for me, but I've taken great pleasure in teaching others to enjoy the benefits of martial arts and fitness training. It has been deeply gratifying to hear back from students, even years later, thanking me for helping them get started on the path to a healthier lifestyle. As much as I've taught my many students, they have also taught me quite a bit. I've had some fabulous teachers both in martial arts and in the fitness industry, so I'd like to thank everyone who has ever spent time on the mats with me in any capacity. Without knowing it, you changed my life.

~Whit McClendon - 2018

Dedication

This book is dedicated to the people out there who are sick and tired of being sick and tired, and are willing to do something about it! I've met and worked with so many folks who want to get in better physical shape but are nervous about getting started because they either don't know what to do or they think that they'll have to kill themselves to get fit. My heart has always gone out to people like that, and I want to help. If this little book can help even a single person to start exercising and live a healthier life, I will have succeeded.

Introduction

Kettlebells have been around for centuries in one form or another. As early as 1000AD in the Sung Dynasty in China, you'll find references to 'stone lock' training, in which stone implements were used in a manner very similar to modern kettlebells. The styles of kettlebell training that are popular today are mostly of Russian origin, and references to strongmen using these iron weights date back to the 1700's.

That said, you don't have to be a Shaolin Monk or a Russian strongman to use kettlebells! Whether you're an experienced athlete or just starting out and learning how to exercise to improve your health, kettlebells can be an effective tool in helping you to reach your goals.

No book can take the place of a human coach that stands right next to you, correcting your form while you train, but since many don't have access to a personal trainer (or the funds to hire one), it is my hope that this book will help you to get started safely. If you have questions after going through the book, feel free to contact me and I'll be happy to help if I can, or point you to additional resources that might be helpful.

In this book, I'll describe and demonstrate some basic kettlebell exercises so that you can see how to perform them yourself. I'll also provide links to videos that will show you the proper technique. Finally, I'll give you some workouts that will help you build strength, burn fat, and improve your overall health if you do them consistently and correctly.

Chapter 1 – Getting Started

In my previous books, I covered some things that anyone should do if they are new to physical training. I'll mention them again here because they're important!

1. **Get a checkup.** If you've been sedentary for a while, it is a good idea to go see your doctor. Let them know that you're going to start a workout program. Hopefully, they'll give you the go-ahead and you can get right to work!
2. **Get some sleep.** Hey, if you're doing regular workouts, you're now an athlete! Your hard-working body is going to need proper sleep so that it can rebuild itself into the one you want. Make sure that you allot enough time each night (or day, if your schedule works that way) so that you can get 7-9 hours of sleep if at all possible. You'll be more alert, and your body will function far better than it would if you were sleep-deprived.
3. **Drink more water!** Most folks I've met and trained are chronically dehydrated, whether they know it or not. The human body is made up of around 65% water...not coffee, juice, or soda. A mere 5% drop in your body's water level can bring about a whopping 30% drop in your work

capacity and mental sharpness! Whoa! It's the kind of thing we all get used to and don't notice the difference until we change it. Yes, you'll go to the bathroom more until your body adjusts, but drinking between 2-3 liters of water a day will help your body become vastly healthier.

4. **Eat the right stuff and avoid the junk.** There are lots of books out there on proper nutrition and hundreds of different approaches to healthy eating. I suggest that you just keep it simple. Eating lean meats and fish, fruits, and vegetables is a good plan. Go easy on the pasta and rice, but that's generally ok too. Eat regular meals and watch your portions. Avoid like the plague anything that you buy from a drive-through, drink water instead of soda, and maybe save the ice cream and cake for one day a week. "You can't outwork a bad eating plan," is a saying that I keep in mind often. It takes over 500 burpees to 'work off' a large order of fries.
5. **Set yourself up to succeed.** Get your favorite music ready to go. Have your workout clothes laid out. Make sure that distractions are kept to a minimum. Make sure you've got a clear space in which to train. If you get everything set up ahead of time,

then you can jump right into your workout without getting bogged down in the other stuff. It's awfully easy to let little obstacles trip you up and help you make the bad decision to skip it 'just for today.'

6. **Don't obsess over the scale.** Please remember that although tracking your weight can be helpful, that number has only a little to do with your overall fitness. It's just a numerical representation of your relationship with gravity. That's it. I have plenty of students who have been training for months to have their scale only move a few pounds down...but they had to buy new clothes because the old ones were hanging on them and their bodies felt like they were new again. Focus on doing the work and being consistent, and don't focus on the scale.
7. **Take rest days.** When you first start exercising, a good schedule is one day of work and then rest the next day. After three workout days, maybe take an extra day off if you need it. Then get back to it! Your body needs rest to recover, so give it the time to do so. I also know of folks who work out almost every single day. I'm one of those, but if I start to feel run-down and unmotivated, I won't hesitate to take a day off. Listen to your body.

OK, now that we've gone over those concepts again, we will talk about the mysterious and often intimidating Kettlebell! Don't let it scare you, though. In time, you will be working out like a champ, getting stronger and fitter before you know it.

Chapter 2 – Kettlebells

Now that kettlebells are so popular, you might run out to your local sporting goods store or hit up Amazon to see what kind of equipment is out there. Brace yourself! There are a ton of them available, some are cheap and some are (whoa!) awfully expensive! Some are well-made and some are absolute junk. Here is what I tell my students to look for if they are planning to purchase their own kettlebells.

1. Classic Style Kettlebells - These are very common, and you can often find these in your local department and sporting goods stores. The lower the weight, the smaller and cuter they are! Their size increases as the weight increases. Some of these are covered with vinyl and might have a rubber pad on the bottom. Those things are not necessary in my eyes, but if buying that kettlebell will get you to start working out, then get it! Price on these can vary greatly, so you'll want to shop around.

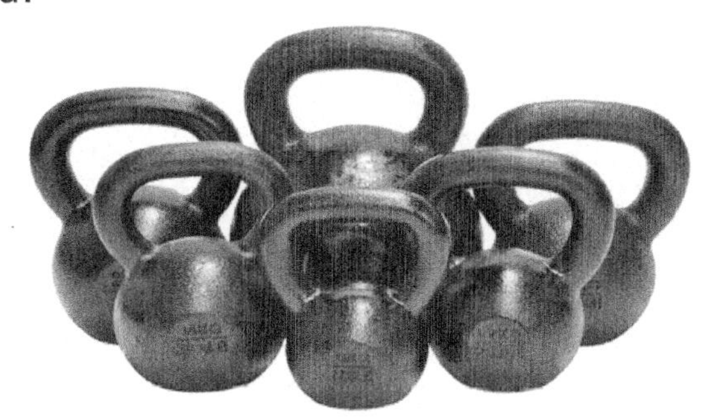

2. Competition Style Kettlebells - These are the type I prefer. Their size and shape are identical, regardless of their weight. They are usually color coded so that you can easily tell the lightest ones from the heaviest, and their handles are more square in shape. These are also called Sport Kettlebells, as they are used for that particular style of lifting and for competitions. The reason I like them is that their size and shape stay the same, so your technique does not change around a larger or smaller kettlebell, only the amount of effort you use.

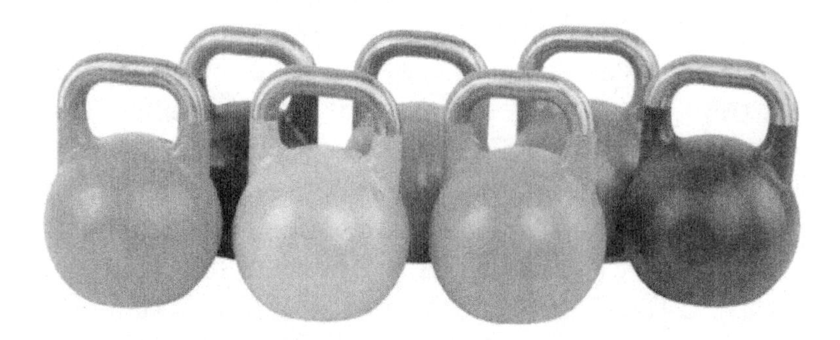

3. Adjustable Kettlebells - These are units in which you can change the weight as desired. It seems like a good idea, but I have my reservations. My suggestion is to avoid adjustable kettlebells and pick a solid bell that is the correct weight for you to start with. That way, you don't have to worry about the adjustable kettlebell coming apart, pinching your skin during certain exercises, or any other mishap that comes along with such things.

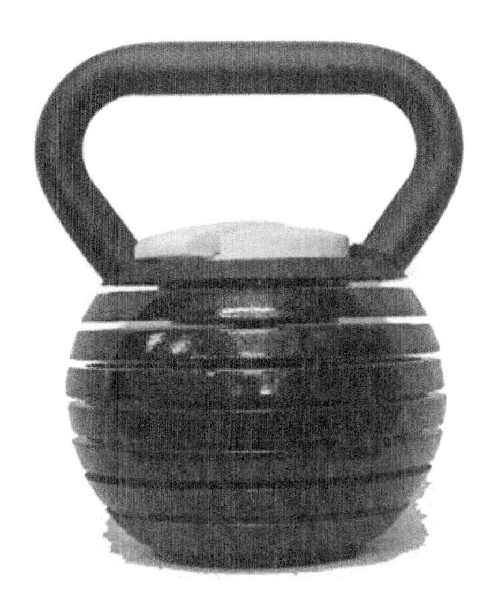

You'll want to find a bell that works best for multiple exercises. That's the beauty of kettlebells...one piece of equipment can be used in so many different ways! If you can press it overhead with one hand without it being too close to the limits of your current strength, then it will probably work for most of the exercises you'll find here. It's often suggested for men to start with a 35 lb/16 kg kettlebell and women to use a 26 lb/12 kg kettlebell, but adjust as necessary and don't go too heavy! You'll get much more out of a kettlebell that you can control, especially when you're just learning the proper exercise techniques.

Chapter 3 – Safety!

First thing's first: you're training with kettlebells so that you get stronger and healthier, NOT so you can hurt yourself! Learning proper technique is essential, and so is warming up thoroughly before you train. Here are a few other rules you should ALWAYS keep in mind when training with kettlebells.

1. Be Aware of your Surroundings – For instance, don't train underneath a low ceiling fan. Be sure that pets and young children will not suddenly try to play with you while you are swinging what is basically a solid iron cannonball around. See that the floor allows good footing, and is not slippery or covered with Legos. If you decide to train outside, then be sure that the sun won't be in your eyes at any time. And if at all possible, train on a surface upon which you can drop your kettlebell in an emergency...without having it crash through the floor to land on your neighbors downstairs.

2. Proper Footwear – Many folks familiar with kettlebell training actually train barefoot so that they can feel the floor beneath them, thus improving balance and coordination. If you must wear shoes, then wear something with a very minimal, flat sole. Giant sneakers are hugely frowned upon, but Chuck Taylors, Vans, wrestling shoes, all of these are often used by kettlebell enthusiasts because they allow the toes to spread out and give a much better sense of the floor.

3. Stay Out of Its Way! - Never contest for space with a kettlebell if it starts to fall or if you 'miss' a rep. Get out of its path! If you try to catch it, you could hurt yourself, so just let it go and get those feet out of the way, too! That means you might not want to work out on your prized wood floor.

4. Use Proper Technique and Procedure - Learn the proper steps for each exercise and follow them carefully! Cutting corners with technique is how injuries happen, so follow the proper steps for each exercise and stay safe. Carefully park the bell after each exercise or set; this means to carefully set it on the ground in a safe manner and place.

5. Warm Up First - Be sure to spend a few minutes oiling your joints and preparing your body for more strenuous exercise. Your workout will be safer, more effective, and more enjoyable if you take the time to warm up well before you get started.

Chapter 4 – Exercises

In this chapter, we're going to go over some fundamental kettlebell exercises that you'll be using in the upcoming workouts. As with any kind of weight-training, the use of correct technique is extremely important, not only so that you can achieve the best possible results from your training, but also for your own safety. In addition to the pictures, there will be links to short videos that show exactly how to perform each exercise correctly.

We will be covering a handful of exercises with some variations in this book. Believe me, if you master these exercises and do them consistently, you'll be well on your way to ferocious fitness!

2-Hand Swings

1. Stand with your feet a little more than shoulder-width apart. Park the kettlebell about a foot in front of you. Bend your knees slightly, and keep your back straight. Reach both hands forward, grip the handle, and tilt the kettlebell towards you.
2. Pull the kettlebell off the ground and 'hike' it between your legs. Your wrists should contact the insides of your thighs very close to your groin. This is the bottom of the swing. Your chest should be pushed forward, your shoulders back, eyes forward.
3. Engage your butt and hamstrings to straighten your legs. Keep your arms loose, engage your lats (back muscles) and swing the kettlebell up to chest height. Keep your shoulders down and back throughout and at the top of the swing. The power actually comes from your lower body here; think of your arms as ropes so you don't pull with them.
4. Hinge at your hips and let the kettlebell swing back between your legs and under your rump, the same position as #3.
5. Repeat step 4 for the next swing.

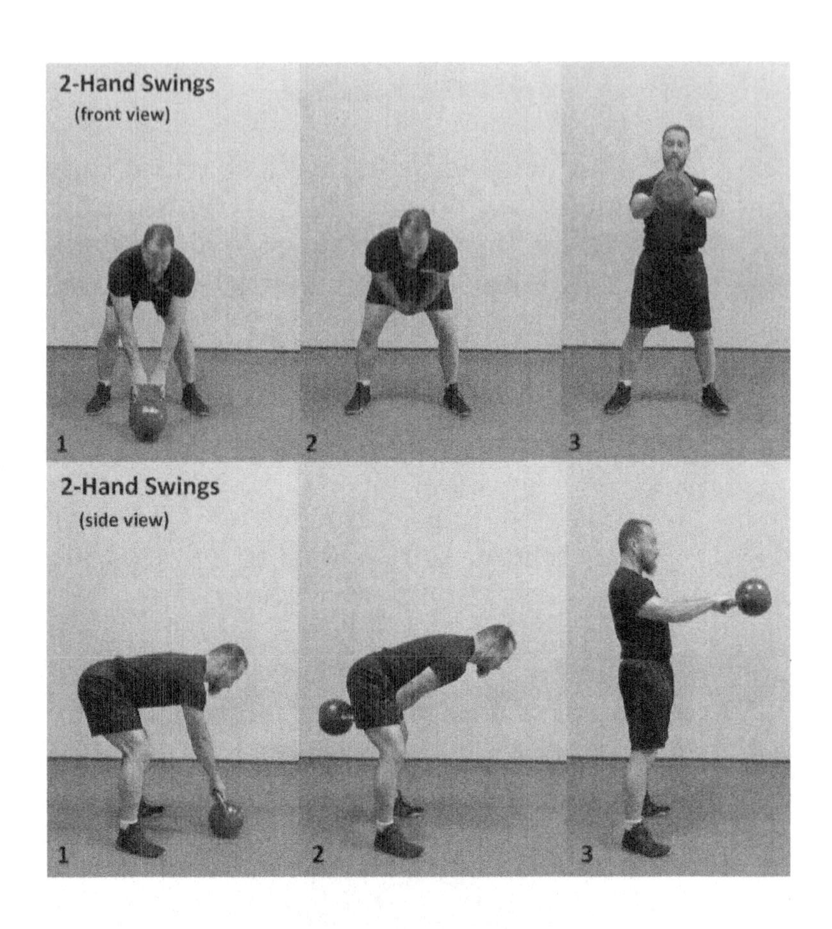

Scan the code for video on Swings!

1-Hand Swings

1. Stand with your feet a little more than shoulder-width apart. Park the kettlebell on the ground foot or so in front of you. Bend your knees slightly, & keep your back straight. Reach one hand forward, grip the handle, & tilt the kettlebell towards you.
2. Pull the kettlebell off the ground and 'hike' it between your legs. Your wrist should contact the insides of your thighs very close to your groin, and your thumb should be pointed behind you. This is the bottom of the swing. Your chest should be pushed forward, your shoulders back, eyes forward. Let the other hand and arm follow along outside your body for balance.
3. Engage your butt and hamstrings to straighten your legs. Keep your arms loose, engage your lats (back muscles) and swing the kettlebell up to chest height. Be sure to square your shoulders, and allow the handle to turn 90 degrees so that it is parallel to the floor. As before, think of your arm as a rope so you don't pull yourself out of alignment.
4. Hinge at your hips and let the kettlebell swing back between your legs and under your rump, the same position as #3.
5. Repeat step 4 for the next swing.

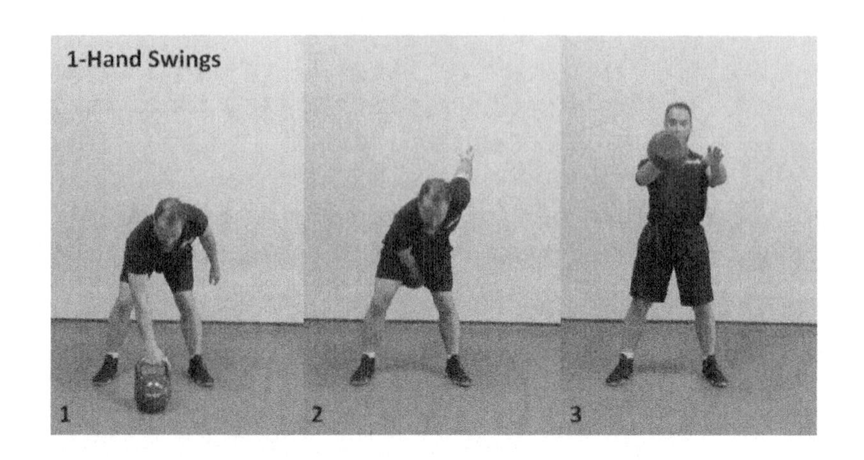
1-Hand Swings
1
2
3

Cleans

In this exercise, you will perform a 1-hand swing at the bottom of the movement, and then bring the kettlebell up to your chest where it will rest in the 'rack position.' This is a great exercise in itself, but is also an integral part of other exercises such as the Clean-and-Press, Clean-and-Jerk, Front Squat, and Thruster, to name just a few.

1. Follow steps 1 through 3 of the 1-Hand Swing.
2. Instead of swinging the bell in front of you at chest height, you will pull it straight up much closer to your body and roll your arm underneath it. Keep your elbow attached to your body.
3. Let the bell come to rest in the crook of your arm, its weight pressing down on your upper chest.
4. Then allow it to roll straight down out of the rack position and hike it underneath your body again, exactly like the bottom of a regular 1-Hand Swing.

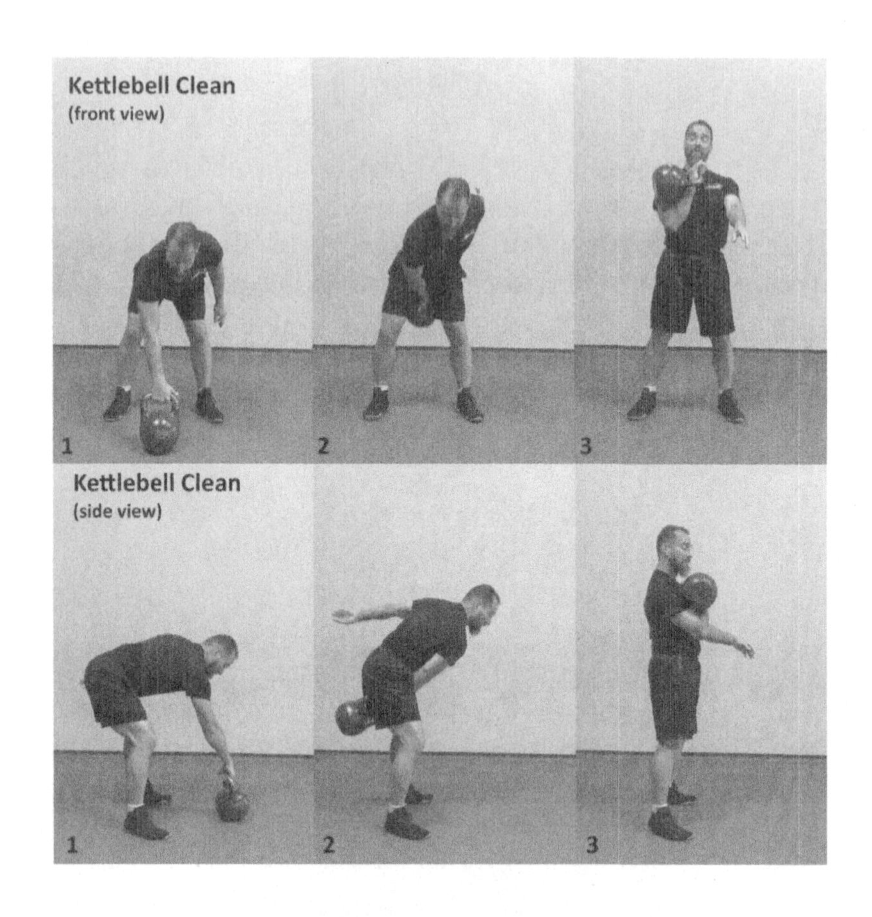

Scan the code for a video on Cleans and the Clean and Press!

Clean and Press

Another great exercise that puts more emphasis on the shoulders!

1. Perform a Clean to get the kettlebell into the rack position.
2. Press the kettlebell directly overhead until your arm is completely straight. Look straight ahead, press your chest forward and your shoulders back.
3. Lower the kettlebell back to the Rack Position.
4. Let the kettlebell roll out of the Rack Position so that you can swing it under your body again for the next repetition.

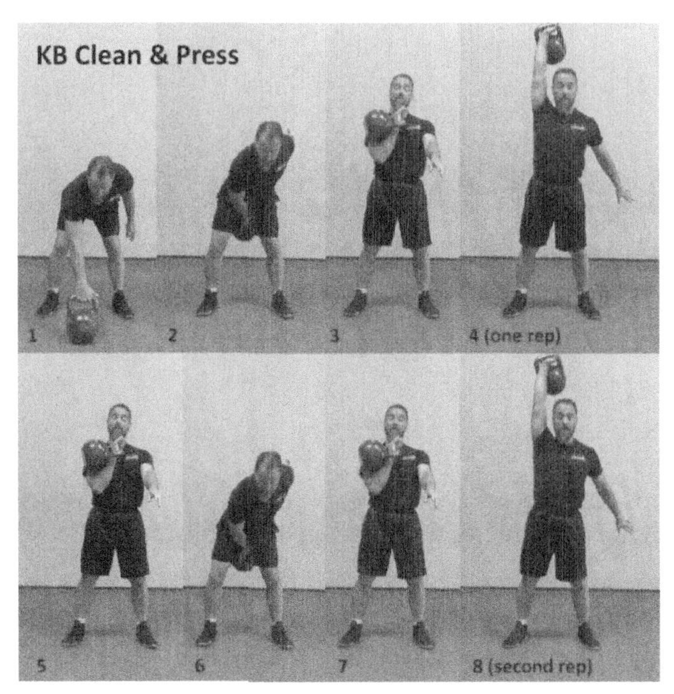

Push Presses

A Push Press brings your legs into the action. You generally can use more weight for this exercise.

1. Clean the kettlebell to the Rack position.
2. Bend your knees slightly.
3. Straighten your legs with power at the same time you press the kettlebell to the overhead position. Remember to keep your arm straight, eyes to the front, and chest out.
4. Lower the kettlebell back to the Rack Position.
5. Repeat steps 2 and 3.

Scan the code for a video on the Push Press!

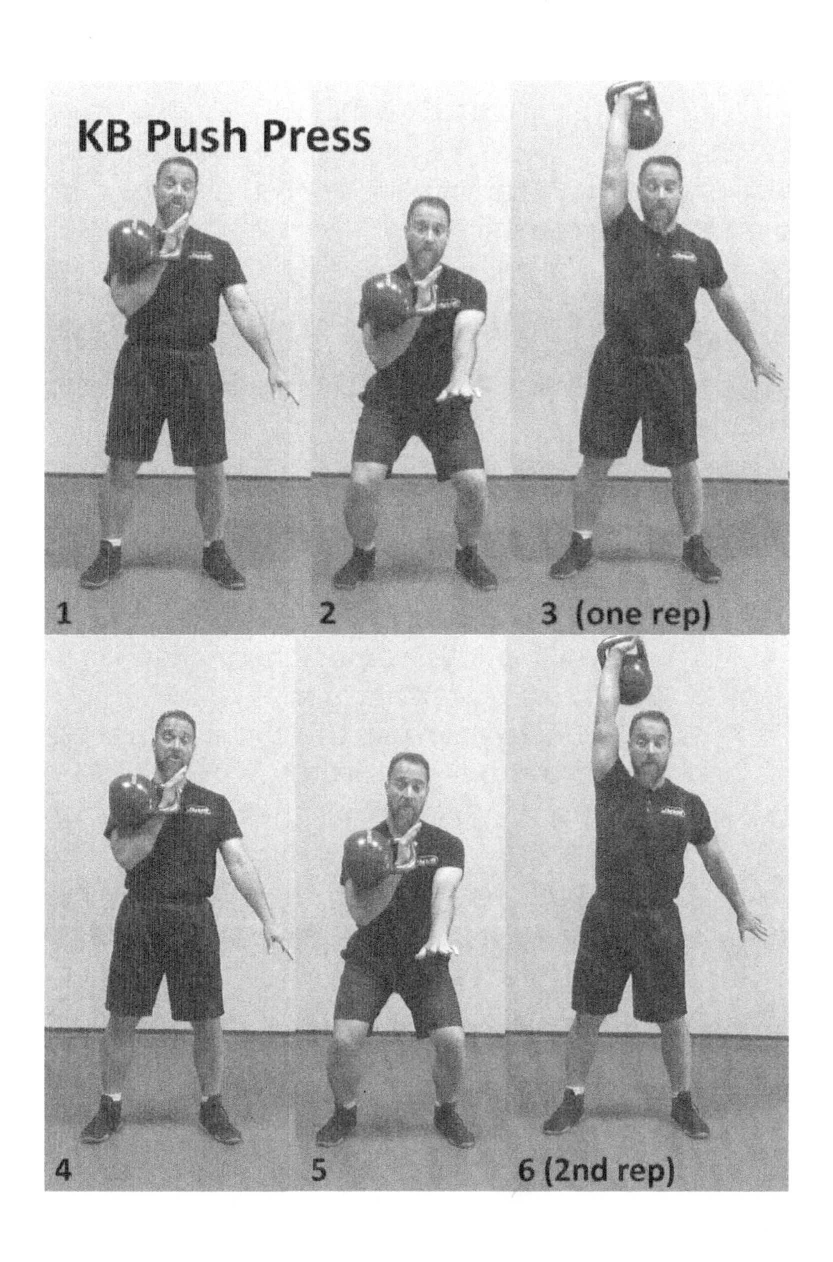
KB Push Press
1
2
3 (one rep)
4
5
6 (2nd rep)

Snatches

Known as The Czar of Kettlebell Exercises, the snatch is a mainstay in any good kettlebell program. It's a unique movement, so take the time to practice it until you can do it well.

The Upward Phase (Getting It Over Your Head!)

1.–2. Follow steps 1 through 3 of the 1-Hand Swing.
3. Forcefully pull the kettlebell up in front of your body. Keep it close to your body, rather than allowing it to swing farther out.
4. Punch your fist through the handle of the bell as it rotates over and on top of your arm as it continues on its way up. It should NOT bang your forearm.
5. Keep the bell moving upwards until it reaches the overhead position.

Scan the code for a video on Snatches!

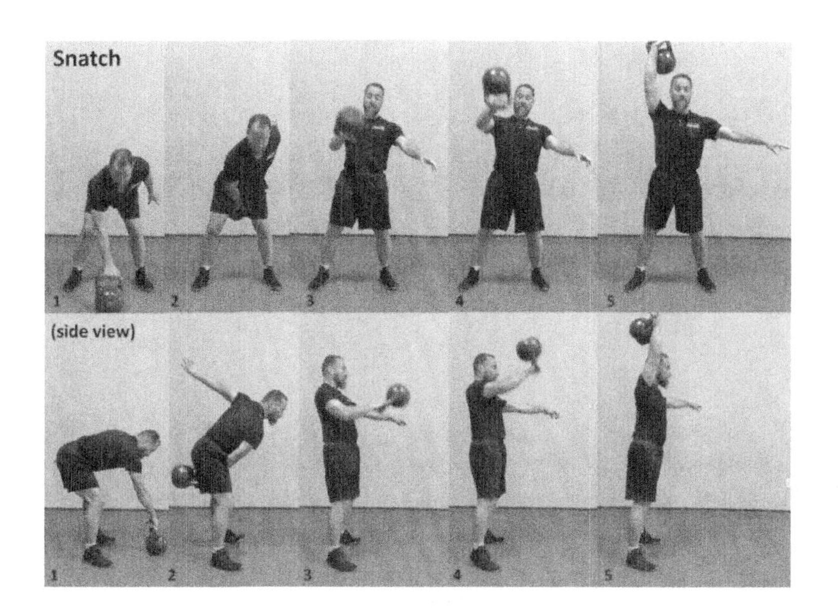

The Downward Phase (Getting It Down From There!)

1. Lean back as you turn your hand palm upwards and twist it so that you allow the kettlebell to descend in front of your body along your centerline. Control the bell as it comes down.
2. Guide it down and into the same hike position you started with.
3. From here, you can continue with additional reps, or just park the kettlebell.

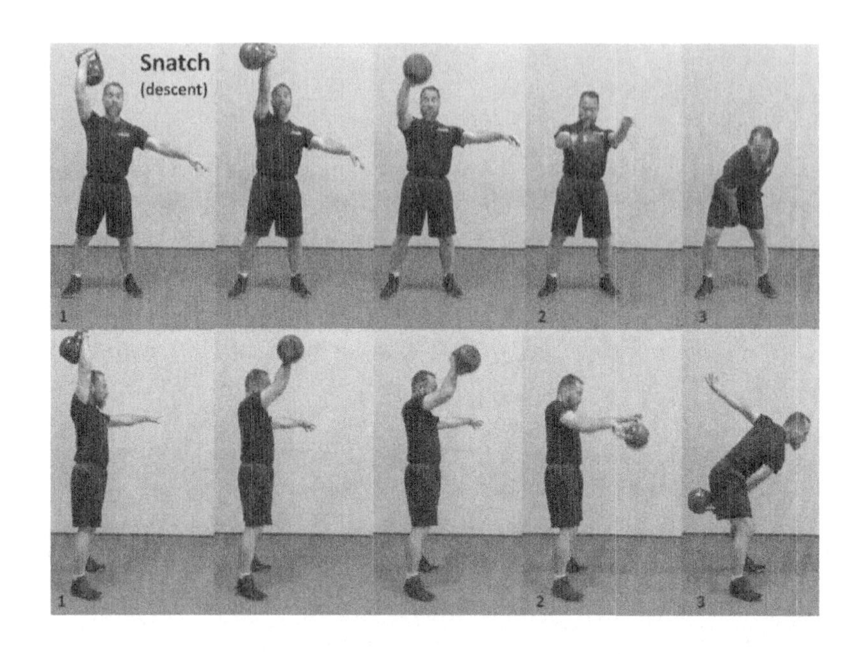
Snatch
(descent)
1
2
3
1
2
3

Turkish Get-Ups

This is one of my all-time favorites. It's also quite challenging, and your body will definitely get stronger after working with these for a while. For the procedure below, I'll be performing the TGU with the right hand.

1. Place your kettlebell on the floor and lie down next to it so that it is on your right side. Roll towards it and into a "fetal" position. Reach your right hand into the handle and grab it, then reach over and put your left hand over your right. Using both hands, pull the kettlebell towards your chest as you roll to your back. Now you're ready to start.
2. Press the kettlebell up towards the ceiling, keeping your knuckles pointed upwards.
3. Drop your left hand and arm to the floor at a 45 degree angle to your body. Straighten out your left leg so it's at the same angle.
4. Punch the kettlebell upwards as you sit up to your elbow, then your hand in one smooth motion.
5. Push into the floor with your left hand and your right foot. Bridge your body up off the floor until it's straight.
6. Pull your left leg back underneath you so you can put your left knee on

the ground directly below your body to support your weight.

7. Remove your left hand from the ground as you straighten your body into a vertical position. The kettlebell should be held directly overhead.
8. Move your left foot so that your lower left leg is in line with the direction your body is facing.
9. Press yourself up to a standing position.
10. Going down is the reverse of going up, one move at a time.

Scan the code for a video on Turkish Get Ups!

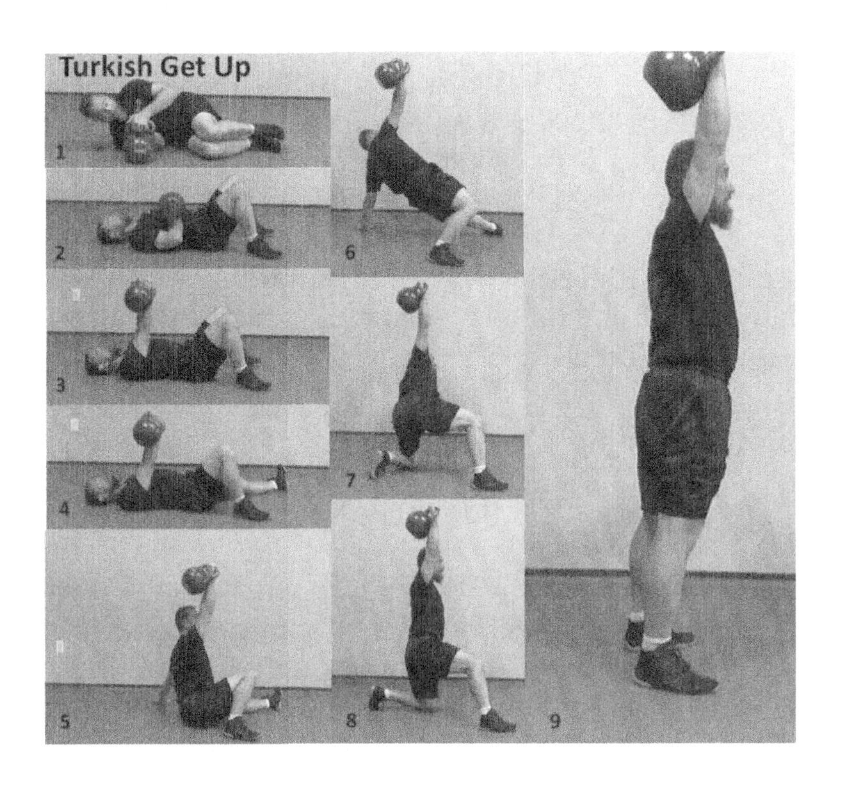
Turkish Get Up
1
2
3
4
5
6
7
8
9

Goblet Squats

This is a great exercise that not only works your legs, but also increases strength in your hands, arms, and shoulders. There are a couple of different ways to hold the Kettlebell during the Goblet Squat: Handle Up, and Handle Down.

1. Stand with your feet shoulder-width apart, holding the Kettlebell at chest height (choose Handle Up or Handle Down method).
2. Inhale as you bend your knees and lower your body into a squatting position, keeping your head and chest upright. Press your knees outwards a bit if they tend to fall inwards as you go down. Strive to get the crease of your hips down below your knees.
3. Return to a standing position, contracting your legs and glutes with a strong exhale.

Scan the code for a video on Goblet Squats!

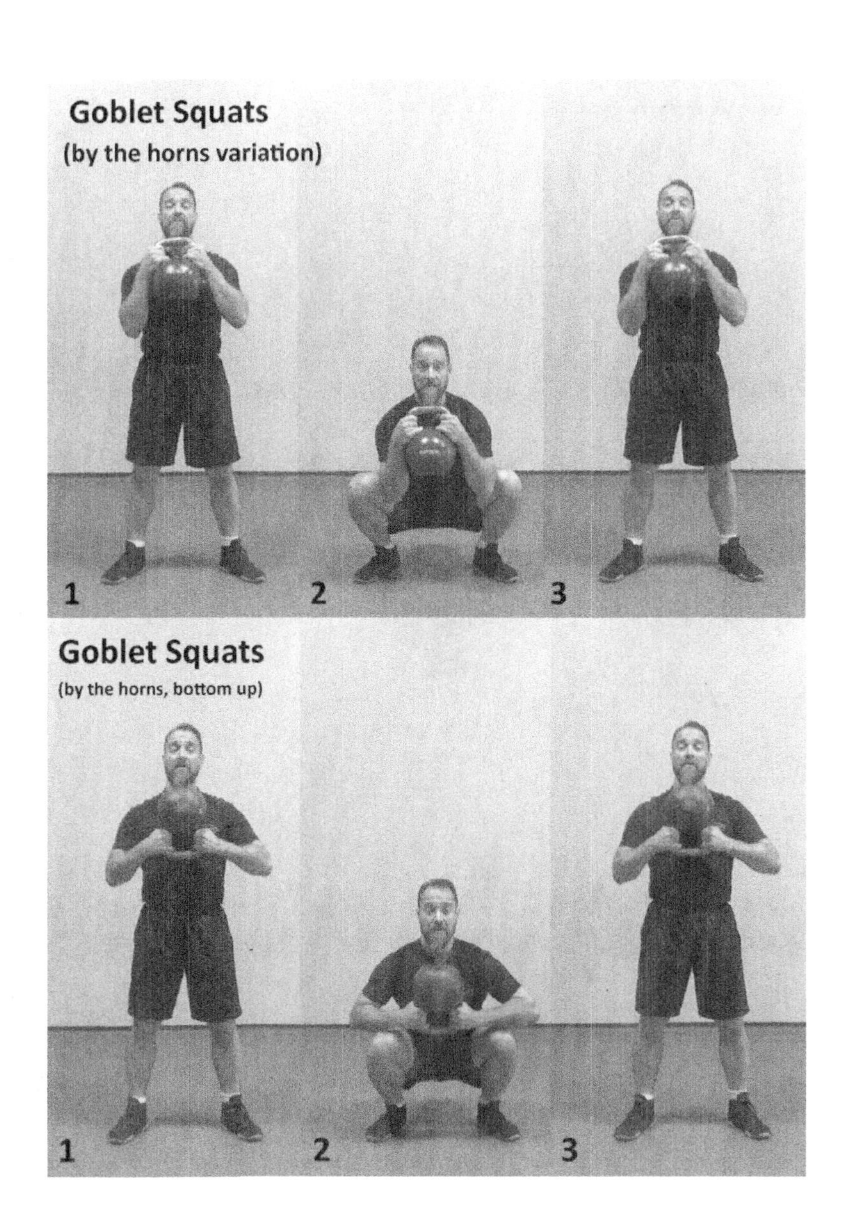
Goblet Squats
(by the horns variation)
1
2
3
Goblet Squats
(by the horns, bottom up)
1
2
3

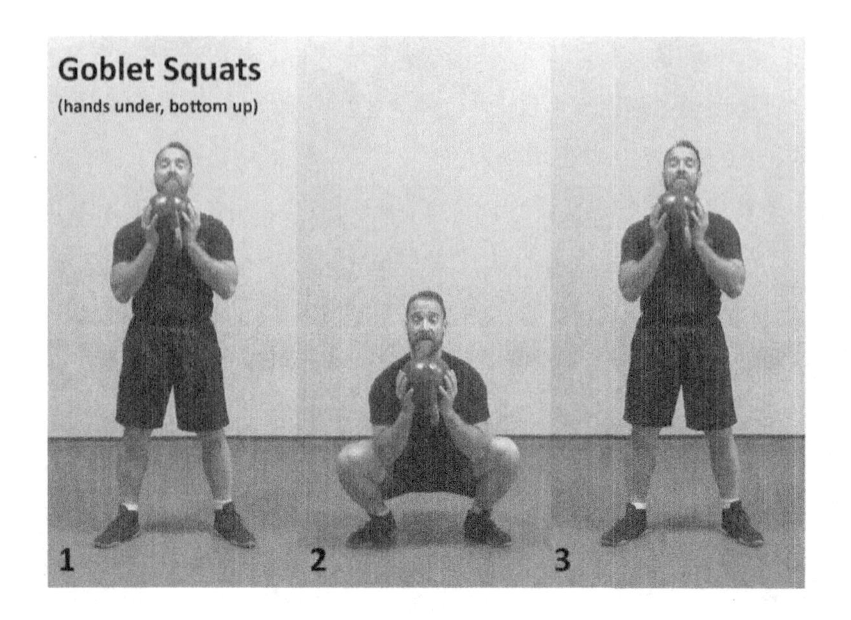
Goblet Squats
(hands under, bottom up)
1
2
3

Chapter 5 – Warm Ups and Workouts

It's very important to prepare your body for strenuous activity, whether you're a beginner about to start your very first workout, or you're an experienced athlete about to do some super-intense training. Either way, it's necessary to get your raise your body temperature and go through a series of motions to prepare your muscles and joints before you train. I often suggest a very easy jog for those who are comfortable running in addition to some basic mobility exercises. Oiling the Joints is a short series of effective movements that get you ready for action.

Oiling the Joints

At Jade Mountain Martial Arts, we have a short set of exercises that we often perform to get our bodies ready to train. We call it "Oiling the Joints." By moving our joints through their range of motion, synovial fluid is pumped into the joints. This lubricates and protects them for more rigorous motions. Our pattern starts at the top of the body and works downwards from there.

Neck: Gently turn your head left and right (as if you're saying 'no') 6 or 8 times. Next, tilt your head back and forth 6 or 8 times (as if you're saying 'yes'). Then tilt it side to side a few times (think of a dog when it hears a funny sound). Last, gently roll it to one side, then to the other.

Shoulders: Roll your shoulders forward a few times, then backwards. Next, twist one arm until your palm faces up, then turn and twist the other arm the same way. (We call it The Egyptian, after the old pictures in the pyramids) Repeat a few times on each side.

Waist: Letting your arms swing, twist your body to the left, then to the right. Repeat 5 or 10 times. Next, rotate your body as if you had a big Hula Hoop, first in one direction a few times, then the other.

Knees: Keep your knees together, and rotate them first one direction a few times, then repeat in the other direction.

Ankles: Trace the outline of one foot on the floor, keeping your knee still. Move first in one direction, then the other. Then repeat with the other foot.

Now that you've Oiled the Joints, it's a good idea to do a few repetitions of the exercises you'll be doing in your workout. Just a few repetitions of each exercise will suffice. Make sure that everything feels good and you're ready to work.

Types of Workouts

There are a few different types of workouts we'll cover in this next section, so let's get to them.

AMRAP

This stands for As Many Rounds (or Repetitions) As Possible. I love running workouts like these because they allow people of very different fitness levels to train simultaneously and everyone gets a great workout! Some super-fit folks might do 15 rounds of work while newer folks might only get 5, but in an AMRAP, everyone gets an opportunity to get a workout that's right for them. Don't worry about keeping up with anyone else, just do what you can do!

X Rounds For Time (RFT)

This stands for a set amount of work that you will try to accomplish. Some folks will complete a workout of 5 rounds of several exercises in just a few minutes, while others take much longer. Either way, you just do what you can do and take note of the time it took you to do it. Remember, the only person you're competing against is the "old you" who didn't work out! Whatever your time is, mark it down, be proud of it, and strive to improve next time.

Circuit

A Circuit is a workout in which you will be doing several different exercises. Starting with one exercise, you will do as many repetitions of that exercises as you can for a set amount of time. Then you switch to the next exercise, and do the same thing. As each time interval passes, you move to the next exercise until you have performed all of the exercises in the workout. That is one round. You can do as many rounds as you decide, or however many the workout calls for.

EMOM

EMOM stands for 'Every Minute on the Minute.' You start the clock and begin your first set. If you complete all the prescribed movements before the end of the minute, you may rest. If not, you start over again at the beginning when the next minute on the clock starts. Continue for however many minutes you decide.

A Word of Caution!!

Whether you're already accustomed to exercising and maybe this is the first time you've decided to try kettlebells, or if you're a total newbie to working out and kettlebells made you want to get started, I want to remind you not to wreck yourself during your first kettlebell workout! Start with a weight that you can control (usually, a 35lb/16kg is common for men and a 26lb/12kg for women, but adjust as necessary!) and be honest with yourself. Learn the exercises with a bell you can actually use, then as you master the movements, you can try something heavier. Don't overdo it! If you feel sharp pains in any of your joints or muscles, or if you start seeing pretty little sparkles in front of your eyes, STOP! Be smart about it. Feel free to contact me if you have any questions, I don't mind a bit.

You'll see other fundamental exercises in the following workouts. If you need a refresher on them, you can find them in Short Workouts for Beginners, the first book in this series.

Now that we've discussed safety and the different types of workouts, let's get started!

WORKOUTS

1. KB Combo #1 (AMRAP) – 10 minutes

10 2-Hand KB Swings
10 Pushups
10 Goblet Squats
10 Situps

Do 10 of each exercise, then move to the next exercise until you've done all four, then start another round. Keep track of how many total rounds you complete, plus how many reps into the final round.

2. KB Circuit #1 (Circuit) – 3-5 rounds

1-Hand Swings (left hand)	1 minute
1-Hand Swings (right hand)	1 minute
Snatches (left hand)	1 minute
Snatches (right hand)	1 minute
Goblet Squats	1 minute

Make it your goal to do each round without stopping and focus on performing good repetitions!

3. KB Fun #1!
(AMRAP) – 15 minutes

3 1-Hand Swings
3 Cleans
3 Push Presses
3 Snatches
3 Goblet Squats
Switch and use other hand

See how many times you can get through both sides of this series in 15 minutes. Rest as little as possible, but as much as you need to.

4. A JMMA Favorite
(RFT) – 1 Round

50/50 1-Hand Swings
16/16 Clean & Presses
30/30 Snatches
30 Goblet Squats

Perform all the reps of each exercise with one hand, then the other, before moving on to the next exercise. Strive to complete each set unbroken, resting in between exercises if necessary.

5. 100 Snatch Test – 5 minutes

Ok, you'll want to be careful of your hands on this one. It's tough. Set your timer and get to work. You can switch hands as often as you like, your goal is to complete 100 snatches within the time limit. If you don't get all 100 snatches done in 5 minutes, just keep going and see how long it takes. Then try and improve on that next time! Good luck!

6. Swings and Pushes (AMRAP) – 10-15 Minutes

10 2-Hand Swings
10 Pushups
10 2-Hand Swings
5/5 Push Presses

Decide on either 10 or 15 minutes, then start the clock. Note how many times you can get through the series.

7. Run, Swing, Burpees! (RFT) – 3 rounds

400m Run
21 2-Hand Swings
15 Burpees

Run through the sequence 3 times, note your time at the end. This is a relatively short workout, so really push to get it done quickly! It may not look like much, but it's a challenge!

8. Tabatas

Tabatas are 4 minute high intensity sets of a single exercise done in a :20 work, :10 rest pattern. That makes 8 rounds of work for each Tabata Interval. As always, warm up thoroughly before you start and be ready to put forth some effort! Try to get as many reps as possible during each :20 burst of exercise. I often suggest that you count the reps on your first interval and try to equal or better that number in the later ones. Here are some Tabata-style kettlebell workouts.

16 minute set
4 Kettlebell Exercises

2-Hand Swings
8 rounds of :20 work, :10 rest = 4 minutes
Snatches
8 rounds of :20 work, :10 rest = 4 minutes
(alternate hands each round)
Clean and Press
8 rounds of :20 work, :10 rest = 4 minutes
(alternate hands each round)
Goblet Squats
8 rounds of :20 work, :10 rest = 4 minutes

In this next workout, you will change exercises for each :20 interval. Start at the top of the list and work your way through the list 4 times.

16 minute set
Mixed Exercises

Exercise	Rest	Work
2-Hand Swings		:20
rest	:10	
Pushups		:20
rest	:10	
Snatches (left hand)		:20
rest	:10	
Snatches (right hand)		:20
rest	:10	
Goblet Squats		:20
rest	:10	
Clean and Press (left hand)		:20
rest	:10	
Clean and Press (right hand)		:20
rest	:10	
Burpees		:20
rest	:10	

Repeat this sequence 4 times.

9. Get Ups and Snatches (RFT) – 1 Round

2 x 5/5 Turkish Get Ups
3 x 10/10 Snatches

Do 5 TGU's on the left side, then on your right, then repeat for another set. Then move to the snatches, doing 10 left, 10 right, then repeating 2 more times. Enjoy!

10. KB Fun #2! (AMRAP) – 15 minutes

1 1-Hand Swing
1 Clean & Press
1 Snatch
1 Goblet Squat

Do all on the exercises on one hand and repeat for a total of 5 times, then switch to the other hand. See how many times you can get through both sides of this series in 15 minutes. Rest as little as possible, but as much as you need to.

11. Swing, Swing, Rest (Circuit) – 15 Rounds

1-Hand Swings (left)	:30
1-Hand Swings (right)	:30
rest	:30

Nothing but 1-Hand Swings in this workout. Set your timer and get to work! Focus on making each repetition as clean and correct as possible, and try to stay steady throughout each set of work.

12. KB Circuit #2 (Circuit) – 5 Rounds

5/5 Clean and Press
5 Goblet Squats
5/5 Get up
15 2-Hand Swings

Do 5 Clean and Presses with one hand, then switch to the other. Then move to Goblet Squats, and so on. Repeat the entire sequence a total of 5 times, noting how long it takes you to complete the all. Rest as little as possible, but as much as you need to.

13. Squats and Swings (EMOM) 15-20 minutes

5 Goblet Squats
15 2-Hand Swings

Start each round at the top of the minute (0:00, 1:00, 2:00, etc), and try to complete all the repetitions before the next minutes starts. If you don't finish in time, simply start over with Goblet Squats when the next minute starts.

14. KB Endurance Workout (AMRAPs) 5 minutes each

2-Hand Swings	5:00
Rest 1:00	
Goblet Squats	5:00
Rest 1:00	
Clean & Press (switch at 5)	5:00
Rest 1:00	
Pushups	5:00
Rest 1:00	
Snatches (switch at 5)	5:00

Perform as many repetitions of each exercise as possible in 5 minutes. Rest for 1 minute, then move to the next exercise. For Clean & Presses and Snatches, switch hands every 5 reps.

15. Burpees and Cleans (RFT) 5 Rounds

10 Burpees
10/10 Cleans

Perform 10 Burpees, followed by 10 Cleans on the left hand, then 10 Cleans on the right hand, and repeat for a total of 5 rounds. Go as fast as possible (with good and safe technique). Rest as little as possible, but as much as necessary.

*   *   *   *

These are all basic workouts that you can use to increase your fitness level while you gain a solid skill base with the kettlebell. As you improve, you might want to try other, more advanced techniques such as using two kettlebells at the same time. Keep your eye out for another book on that subject from me!

Chapter 6 – Hand Care

Taking care of your hands is vital when you start working with kettlebells. This kind of activity is going to produce calluses over time, and if you don't know how to deal with them, then it's likely that they will grow to the point that they may rip, which will set you back in your training. Nobody wants that! Start slowly, and remember that even if you're strong enough to keep lifting, it's a bad idea to continue if your hands are getting damaged.

If you start to feel a tear coming on, then STOP. There's nothing smart about wrecking your hands so you can finish your set or workout only to find that you can't train for days until they heal.

When calluses start to form, that's good! It's your body getting conditioned to your new activity! But as I mentioned, you don't want them to go untended so they tear during your kettlebell work. That hurts.

So what's the solution? I prefer using an emery board to simply smooth them out so that they never get large enough to be pulled off. A pumice stone in the shower also works, you just use the stone to smooth out the calluses while you sing your favorite song (OK, singing is optional). One product I've used to keep my hands in good shape is Working Hands Hand Cream. When my hands start getting too rough, I use this stuff just before I got to sleep at night. Just rub it into your hands and forget about it. Easy! There are other lotions (I've heard Corn Huskers Lotion mentioned more than once by kettlebell enthusiasts) but this works well for me, and it doesn't feel greasy.

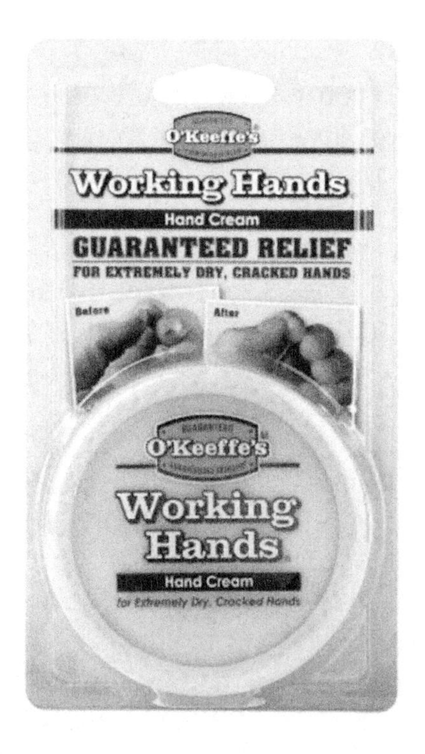

I generally don't recommend gloves because they often cause additional friction when working with kettlebells, causing blisters rather than preventing them. Also, it's harder to feel the handle of the bell through a glove.

It's better to start with light kettlebells and work yourself gradually up to heavier bells and harder workouts so that your hands get conditioned without injury.

Chapter 7 – Summing It Up

Ok, now you have more of a gameplan than you had before! You've got a handful of fundamental exercises and some good, solid workouts than can whip you into shape. Hopefully, I have provided clear instructions that will help you get started with kettlebells. Like any exercise program, you need to be consistent and give it some time so you can see and feel your results. Be patient, and just do what you can. Choose a kettlebell that fits you, and train 3 to 5 times a week until it just feels too light. You might be surprised at how quickly you start thinking of getting a heavier bell! If you have questions, don't be afraid to contact me. I love helping people and offering support, so don't be shy. Give me a holler and let me know how you're doing!

1. **Choose a kettlebell you can handle.**
2. **Start out easy.**
3. **Schedule workouts ahead of time.**
4. **Clean up your eating.**
5. **Drink more water.**
6. **Take rest days!**
7. **Just keep at it. Be determined, and do your best!**
8. **Ask for help when you need it. (I'm just an email away!)**

Follow these steps and watch your health improve. You can do this! The fact that you're reading this book tells me that you're already headed in the right direction. I hope you enjoy working with kettlebells as much as I do, and thank you for picking up this book...now go get to work!

The End

Get the other books in the Jade Mountain Workout Series!

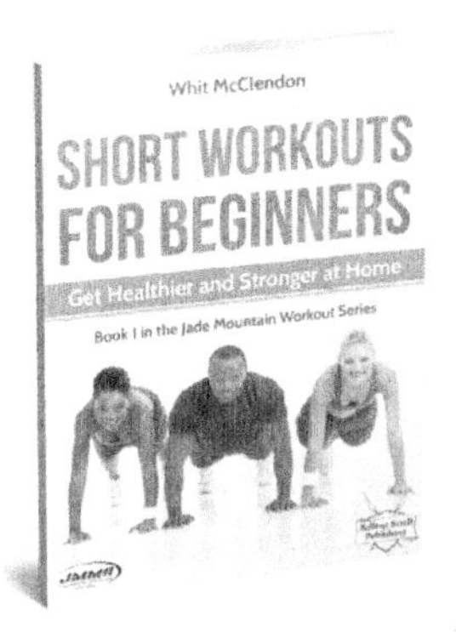

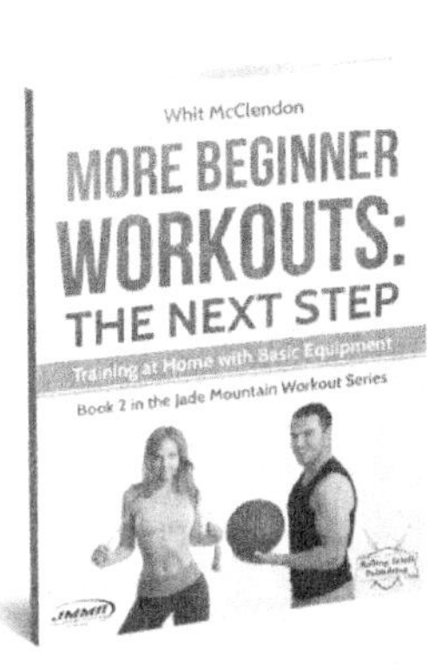

If you're ready to get fit and improve your health, then these books are for you! You can get fitter and stronger than ever just by exercising at home. No more expensive gym fees, no more taking the time to drive to the gym, you'll be on your way to better strength and fitness in the comfort of your own home! Don't like the music the gym has playing? This book lets you choose when and where you exercise, and YOU pick the tunes!

These books cover specific exercises and provide detailed instructions on how to do them correctly and safely. In addition, you'll find simple, easy-to-follow workouts that can help you lose weight and gain strength, all on your own. Included are links to videos so that you can see exactly how to perform the movements properly.

Available in paperback and e-book!

Amazon US:

Amazon UK:

About The Author

Sifu Whit McClendon was born on October 31, 1969 in Freeport, Tx. He grew up in Angleton Texas and was active in martial arts, track and field, and playing the clarinet in band. After working in the petrochemical field as a CAD drafter for many years, Whit finally realized his life's dream of becoming a full-time martial arts instructor. He now lives with his family in Katy, Texas, plays lacrosse as often as possible, and runs Jade Mountain Martial Arts.

Whit has intensively studied Kung Fu, Krav Maga, Taiji, Kickboxing, and Brazilian Jiu Jitsu since 1982. He has been a CrossFit Lvl 1 certified Coach, an HKC and level 2 IKFF Kettlebell instructor, and is well-versed in the techniques and applications of cardio & resistance training. He is a CrossFit Games competitor, a 2 time National AAU Shuai Jiao silver medalist, a Tough Mudder enthusiast, lacrosse player, and a 4 time Houston Half-Marathon Finisher.

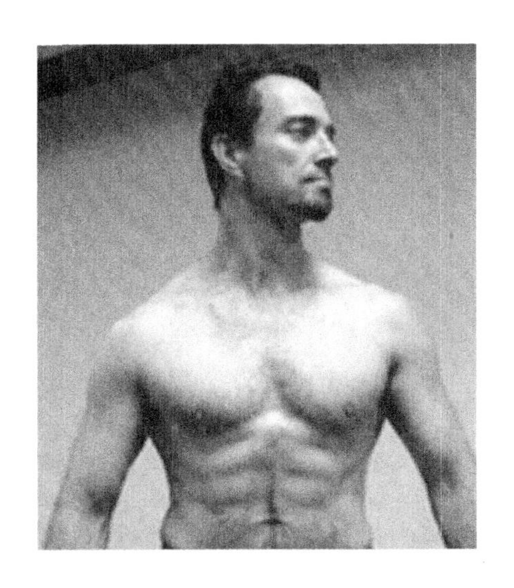

whitmcc@jmma.org
www.jmma.org
www.whitmcclendon.com

Printed in Great Britain
by Amazon